Parkinson's Caregivers:

Yes, There is Hope!

Parkinson's Caregivers: Yes, There is Hope!

Cheryl Hughes

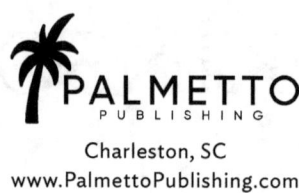

Charleston, SC
www.PalmettoPublishing.com

Parkinson's Caregivers

Copyright © 2023 by Cheryl Hughes

All rights reserved

No portion of this book may be reproduced, stored in a retrieval system, or transmitted in any form by any means–electronic, mechanical, photocopy, recording, or other–except for brief quotations in printed reviews, without prior permission of the author.

First Edition

Paperback ISBN: 979-8-8229-1835-1

eBook ISBN: 979-8-8229-1836-8

This book is dedicated to my friends and fellow caregivers of the Parkinson's Support Group of Peachtree City, Georgia.

Thank you for your encouragement and support for my blog and for this book.

I hope this book brings you hope.

Don't give up, dear friends. The long days and longer nights are worth it.

Thank You

To my daughters, Margie and Audrey, my sons-in-law, Walter and Charles, and to my 7 grandchildren. You were right here with me every step of the way. I could not have cared for Carlton without each of you. Thank you for visiting often, for including Carlton in your lives, for walking slowly to match his speed, and for pushing the wheelchair for me. To my grandchildren, I love that you have learned compassion early in life. I love you all.

To Nurse Rachel for her care for Carlton and me during those long Hospice days and nights through COVID-19. (It was months after meeting her before I ever saw the bottom half of her face! Masks were mandatory.) You helped me through those dark days, and you gave me a greater appreciation of the "thin place" as Carlton left this earth for Heaven. You prayed with me, cried with me, and loved both of us through those final days of Carlton's life here on earth. Thank you for writing chapter 3 of this book with me.

To Franck, our dedicated CNA. You took extraordinary care with Carlton to make him feel special and important. But thank you most of all for helping us navigate those hallucinations and for calming Carlton's fears of the "men with guns" outside the door. You prayed with us and quoted Scripture with us, and your calming influence eased our fears. Thank you for being there when we needed you.

Introduction

My husband, Carlton Hughes, had Parkinson's Disease for about 23 years, and I was his caregiver. I am writing this book during the first year after his passing, and looking back it seems that in many ways those years have flown by. And yet, sometimes the clock seemed stuck. This book is specifically about how to have hope while caring for a loved one with Parkinson's Disease. However, many things in the book apply to those with other diseases, especially neurological diseases.

Even though caring for him was one of the hardest things I have ever done, watching his health decline and his body waste away near the end, was even harder. Looking back, I do not regret my decision to care for him at home, and I'm thankful my good health enabled me to spend that time with him. But whether at home or in a facility, you are still the one who cares. That makes you their advocate and caregiver.

This book is my gift to you, dear caregiver. I know that your care for your loved one is your labor of love. Knowing how hard you work and what you give up daily, I hope my words encourage you to stay the course. Don't give up. Caring for your loved one is a sacred task, no matter what form it may take. May God give you the strength and the faith that you need.

Contents

Dedication vii

Thank You ix

Introduction xi

CHAPTER ONE *The Diagnosis* 1

CHAPTER TWO *Living With It* 23

CHAPTER THREE *Advanced Parkinson's Disease* 49

CHAPTER FOUR *Hospice Care* 65

CHAPTER FIVE *What I Learned From Caregiving* 79

Chapter One
The Diagnosis

I wish I had gone with him to that doctor's appointment. I should have gone with him, but we had no idea that the diagnosis would be Parkinson's disease. That was not even on our radar. My husband, Carlton, had symptoms that were not what we associated with Parkinson's (PD). He didn't really shake, and that's what we thought PD was all about.

His symptoms seemed random to us, and we never connected the dots in a way that came up with a picture of PD. This is how it happened.

The first two things he noticed were that when he walked, his left arm did not swing as usual and his steps were becoming shorter. He noticed these things because he took public transportation partway to work each day, and from the train station he walked about a fourth of a mile on a sidewalk. He noticed the length of his steps first because the sidewalk was composed of sections of concrete, all the same size. At first, he walked about four steps in each section, but over the course of a few months he noticed he was now taking almost seven steps in each section of the sidewalk. We talked about it one night over dinner. A few weeks later he mentioned that his left arm didn't swing. He could make it swing consciously for a few minutes, but as soon as his focus was on something else, his arm ceased to swing.

There were two more symptoms that propelled him to see a doctor, which he seldom did. A close friend asked him to play the organ for her wedding, and he was honored to be asked. He was a professional musician, so he felt very competent for this task. However, he had not played in public for about a year, so he practiced in earnest. As I listened to him play, I noticed a difference in the quality of his playing. When I asked him about it, he said the right and left hands just were not in sync. He was certain that a little more practice would make the difference. He even mentioned this to a close musician friend, and he thought the same thing. But practice did not make a difference, and soon it was evident there was something wrong. His left hand was slow and clumsy, which was very troublesome to us both.

The final symptom that sent him to the doctor was an observation I made one day as I was walking behind him. From the back, he looked like someone who had just had a stroke. He was hugging his left arm to his body, and his left leg was dragging slightly. When I walked up beside him, I said, "You're right. Something is wrong with your left side. You need to go to a doctor!"

But neither one of us connected these symptoms to Parkinson's disease. And we were not prepared for the way the doctor delivered the news. He was a general practitioner who had never seen Carlton before. After listening to Carlton describe his symptoms and observing him, he said, "Sir, I don't know you, but by the description of your symptoms and looking at your face, I can tell that you have Parkinson's disease."

When he first heard the diagnosis, Carlton was stunned, shocked, and almost horrified. Even when he told me that night, neither of us realized the ramifications of the doctor's words, nor could we fathom the scope of Parkinson's disease. In some respects, we wished we had not gotten a diagnosis because it changed the way we were thinking. But not knowing would not have helped the situation. Having a name for the condition allowed us to focus on helping my husband. The diagnosis was not a death sentence. It was a prescription for how to live the rest of our lives. Looking back, we realized that having a diagnosis was a good thing.

Do We Need a Diagnosis?

It is true that there are pros and cons about receiving such a devastating diagnosis. One of the cons is that we tend to think about the future differently. We might even think about the end of life more often than we did previously. This is normal but not healthy. Having a diagnosis just means that we vaguely know the underlying cause of the health problems we may face going forward. We just don't usually think about life in those terms. With the diagnosis of a degenerative disease, we understand that our condition will deteriorate at a rate that is probably more rapid than aging in general. So, we begin watching for signs. For me, it felt like I was always waiting for the other shoe to drop. I was always waiting for the next problem, the next health issue, wondering if it was caused by Parkinson's.

Another con is that we blame everything on Parkinson's. Every time a new problem arises, we wonder if it is a result of PD, or the medication to control the PD. That might cause us to run to the neurologist, thinking it is related to PD, when it is really related to another organ of the body. And we might postpone going to a specialist who might be better equipped to treat this symptom.

However, there are even more pros for having a diagnosis. Not knowing what is physically wrong with our loved one is terrifying. Our imagination runs wild if we let it, and we sometimes jump to the "worst case scenario." Just ask someone who has struggled for years to find their underlying problem. This causes anxiety, fear, and worry. Having a diagnosis means we KNOW what is happening under the skin, at least in general. Putting a name to a disease or condition brings clarity for the treatment. It gives direction to the entire family. It also means we can research, we can look online for information, we can read books about it, we can identify with others who have it, we can choose doctors who specialize in this disease, and we can join support groups where we will find help and encouragement.

In all our research, we must remember this fact—our loved one will not have every symptom we read about. He/she may not have them in the same order as the research indicates, and the severity may be different than described. Pre-existing conditions influence the scale of each symptom as well as the timing.

There used to be no definitive test to confirm a PD diagnosis, except an autopsy. However, there are several methods used today to confirm a diagnosis of Parkinsonism or a variation thereof. One is a DAT scan, which can help verify or identify various markers. It is also widely believed that if the patient responds positively to Carbidopa/Levodopa (C/L), a diagnosis of Parkinson's is correct. This is an over-simplification of the diagnosis process, but it provides a place to begin. It is best to consult a neurologist who has experience with Parkinson's.

One more quick note about doctors and diagnosing. There are several types and variations of PD, and many times doctors diagnose one type. But over time after observation, they realize their diagnosis was slightly off, and there is a variation at work in the patient. So, it isn't surprising when the doctor alters the diagnosis on the second or third visit. If the diagnosis is a type of Parkinsonism or something related, much of the information in this book will still apply.

But I'm getting ahead of myself. Knowing is better than wondering because it gives us focus. We can concentrate on things that will help when we know the problem. It gives direction for treatment. So, we can be thankful when we have a diagnosis.

COMMON SYMPTOMS

What drove us to make the appointment with the doctor? What were the early symptoms? Looking back, I believe it took us several months of noticing symptoms before we felt they were serious enough for my husband to see his doctor. Many PD patients will say they had the disease long before they were ever diagnosed.

In general, my husband had very few things wrong with him other than common ailments like high blood pressure (but not TOO high) and high cholesterol (but nothing to worry about since he was taking medication). He had never had problems with his heart, but his father died after his third heart attack, so the doctor kept a close eye on his heart health.

Earlier in this chapter, I described some of the symptoms that prompted him to go to the doctor, but others were beginning to appear as well. The truth is this: there is no "regular" order in which the myriad of Parkinson's symptoms will appear. Parkinson's disease affects every part of the body, so the early symptoms can manifest anywhere. Any of these could show up first: double vision, blurry vision, handwriting that becomes smaller and smaller, stumbling, sudden lack of facial expression, slowed walk or speech, suddenly softer speech, and even cognitive decline.

Doctors have differing opinions on which symptoms are the result of Parkinson's. However, through the Michael J. Fox Foundation for Parkinson's Research, it has been proven that these symptoms and many more are common in PD patients. Some symptoms alert us to the presence of the disease while others are side effects of medication used to control it. The question I asked most often during the years I cared for my husband was this, "Is this new symptom part of Parkinson's disease?" Opinions among medical professionals vary so much that eventually I stopped asking and just assumed that it was.

Now that we have the diagnosis, what should we do as we leave the doctor's office? We may receive a brochure about the disease, and that is helpful. But sometimes we don't really know what to do next. Here are some suggestions.

What to Do After Receiving the Diagnosis

After the initial shock of the doctor's news wears off, we must decide how to tell the world around us. Disclosing this news should be done on our timetable. And whenever possible, the wishes of our loved one, the patient, should be honored. In fact, going forward, it is helpful to ask their opinion and think about each situation from their perspective.

Families are complicated, so there is no formula that works in every situation. But here are some things to consider when respecting the dignity of our loved one and the privacy of our family.

First, we can consider keeping the diagnosis in the immediate family for a short period of time. Close family members may need time to process the news before announcing it to the larger circle of friends and family. Most likely we will tell our life partner first (if they were not with us), but then the decision must be made concerning when to tell our children, especially young children, parents, siblings, other relatives, close friends, casual acquaintances, friends at work, clubs, churches, and schools. The list is extensive!

In today's society, once a few people know, it will be difficult to control the narrative, especially due to social media. It might be wise to develop a family-wide standardized statement to be used on all platforms and in all announcements. We should also craft appropriate responses to questions that will be inevitable. For instance, some might ask about our loved one's current symptoms of PD. In response we might choose a few symptoms to mention. There is no need to list everything. Others might ask about life expectancy. A common answer would be, "This is our time to live, not to think about the END of life." When pressed with those questions, different family members might give different information or a different response, so it is wise to talk about them in a family meeting.

Second, before announcing it to the next layer of friends, it is important to understand the disease overall. That information can be found online, in books, in brochures from your doctor, or from friends who have already been diagnosed. People are going to expect us to know about the disease in general. And if they ask a question to which we do not know the answer, we can ask them to research it, or write it down so we can look it up later. But we will want to have a cursory knowledge of the disease as soon as possible. It is important to remember and point out to friends and family that all patients are different and will have slightly different symptoms and issues and timetable. The severity of each symptom also differs from patient to patient. This is due to pre-existing conditions, body type, genetics, environment, attitude (mental health), etc. So, when someone asks, "Well, my uncle had Parkinson's and he _____. Why doesn't your husband/wife do that?" We can simply answer that "everyone is different, and PD presents itself differently in each person."

As friends and family hear about the diagnosis, some will voice their willingness to help, both now and in the future. They will become our support network. Some may be overzealous and want to offer advice and opinions. We can listen and even take mental notes, but we don't have to act on them until we have investigated their merits. And there will be others, even family, who will drift away and keep their distance.

It was eye-opening for me to see the different reactions of family and friends when we announced Carlton's diagnosis. Looking back, I can see the three categories of responses—those who leaned in to be there for us the entire twenty-three years, those who were there when I contacted them, and those who really didn't want to see how much he was changing. For some of them, it hurt too much to watch. I had to learn to accept each group without judgment.

Third, plan ahead. This is a good time to begin to think about getting our home ready for our loved one as their mobility changes. There are many websites to give you suggestions, and we will include some in the following chapter.

Besides getting our physical home ready, it's time to begin to get our finances arranged for the future. If our loved one has overseen the payment of bills, it's time for the caregiver to be introduced to that part of life and gradually take on that task when it becomes necessary. This includes knowing about passwords and insurance policies as well.

One of the best things we did at this stage was seek the advice of an attorney who specializes in estate planning or elder law. This is the time to prepare for our financial future specifically. We do not know how long any of us have on this earth, so we should consider this a wake-up call concerning getting our paperwork in order—wills, advanced medical directive, life insurance, power of attorney, etc. It's best to schedule it now, especially if there's already cognitive decline. During the next few months, we should try to work in some time for honest conversation about how we want to live out our final days on earth, and an attorney can guide us in that process. When we begin discussing end-of-life issues, the conversation might seem stilted or forced. But gradually, over time and with practice, talking about death and funerals and caskets should become easier, both with our loved one and family.

Lastly, this is the healthiest our loved one may be (in general). For that reason, this could be the best time to travel and visit friends and family. We cannot put this off for the future. Our best days are probably right now, so let's take advantage of today.

Mental Health

Each of us responds differently to a diagnosis, and for some it is devastating. For those who already struggle with depression or anxiety, this diagnosis can magnify those feelings. Thankfully, there are several ways to cope with those feelings of despair. Seeking the help of a professional like a counselor or psychologist can be helpful when we are honest with them about our feelings and the reasons for them.

Since Parkinson's is a neurological disease, it is best to find a good neurologist, and he/she can help if we tend toward depression. Admitting that we need help at the outset will prevent problems along the way. However, if we ignore our feelings, they will compound over the course of the disease, and the saddest part is that there is a way to prevent depression. So, it is better to address this with our doctor early after the diagnosis. Just taking a pill like an anti-depressant can make a huge difference in our outlook for the future.

There are two other areas that will help with mental health. The first is exercise. Most of us agree that exercise is important for mobility, but we might not think of it in conjunction with maintaining mental wellness. Regarding degenerative disease, science has proven that exercise—even slight exercise—provides the body with positive mental health.

Finally, exercising our faith will give us a positive outlook on life, even while we're challenged with a degenerative disease. Whatever our faith and however strong it is, the community and the catechism of our faith will give us strength to persevere in the days to come. This is the time to lean into that faith.

A Medical Notebook

Now is the time to keep a medical notebook to take with you to every doctor visit, not just the neurologist appointments. Before this diagnosis, there might have been no reason to write things down because many adults visit a doctor only once a year and have no major issues. So, there may have been fewer reasons to take notes. But now, that has suddenly changed. It is very important to have a notebook/journal because there will suddenly be many things to remember. The format is totally up to you, but here are some things to include in it:

- A business card from each doctor you see, even if you only see them once
- A separate page for each visit where you notate the following:
    - Blood pressure
    - Weight
    - Pulse/oxygen

- Problems you spoke with the doctor about
- Problems the doctor noticed
- New medication names and dosage
- Any side effects the doctor mentioned to watch for
- Anything the doctor asked you to watch for before the next visit
- Any suggestions the doctor gave you to help at home

Some doctors will print out some of this information and hand it to you at the end of the visit, so keeping a loose-leaf notebook to put them in is also an option. In between visits, you can also write down any questions that you want to ask the doctor at the next visit. Also note changes in your loved one and write the date you first observed it. That will be important information for the doctor.

Aside from the medical journal, we found it was helpful to keep a digital copy on the computer of my husband's medications so that it could be easily changed when needed and easily printed before the next visit to any type of physician. Beside the name of the medication, we noted the doctor who prescribed it, the strength of the medication, and how many times a day he took it.

Keeping a copy to hand to the nurse or doctor means that we do not have to recall the medications or write them all down at each visit. The caveat is that we are responsible to update the digital version each time medications change. But it is worth that inconvenience in the long run.

List of Medications:

Name of Drug	Strength (mg)	Dosage (times daily)	Prescribing Doctor
Medication name			

Medications

It is not my place to recommend or prescribe medications because that is best left to the physicians. However, there are some important things to know about medications that are unique to Parkinson's disease.

Currently your loved one may be managing his/her own medications and doing well taking them on time and in the correct dosage. It is likely that over time, you as the caregiver will have to take on that responsibility because of their decline in mobility or cognition. By paying attention to names of drugs that your loved one takes, you may eliminate many problems or mistakes in the future. You may also hear about specific drugs on television, read about them online, or hear about them from a friend, and you will need to research them to see if they are appropriate for your loved one. Yes, this used to be the task of the physician, but society has changed over the years, and it is now incumbent on the consumer/patient/caregiver to do their own preliminary investigation into medications.

It is common for physicians to encourage their patients to take new or experimental drugs. To encourage that, many pharmaceutical companies visit physicians and elicit their business by providing lunch for their office staff and giving them free samples of the drug they are promoting. It is a good practice to research each new prescription before filling it. Look for side effects, benefits, availability, and cost. Sadly, many new drugs are extremely expensive, even after insurance. However, there are sometimes ways to make these drugs affordable. Check with your doctor, their office staff, your pharmacist, and the website for the specific drug and/or disease. There are several websites that direct the consumer to grant programs designed for specific illnesses. It is entirely possible to obtain medications for very little cost or even free. Remember that drug companies need patients to take their products, so they are willing to help with the cost. Don't be afraid to ask for help in this.

Specific disease support group meetings are another resource to find out more information about medications, including common side effects (very important) and financial aid to pay for them. Sometimes groups bring in speakers to introduce the group to new drugs that have become available. Attending those might give you an opportunity to ask questions about a new medication.

One other valuable resource can be your pharmacist. If possible, develop a working relationship with your local pharmacist early after diagnosis. They will be communicating with your doctors during this journey each time you need a prescription refilled, and they will be supplying you with each new medication you try. When your doctor prescribes a medication that is newly marketed, you will need to talk with your pharmacist about accessibility to the drug.

At our pharmacy, which is in a large grocery store chain, my husband was the only patient on a particular PD drug at first. That means that this was not a drug on the regular supply list. The pharmacist had to ask for it specifically and show that there was an actual customer requesting it. Thankfully, I already had a working relationship with that pharmacist, so it was not a problem to get the drug. Our pharmacists have been personally involved in my husband's care, and for that I am very thankful.

On a personal note, our insurance company has tried to pressure me into using a mail-order prescription drug service, but I have resisted for two reasons. The first involves the personal relationship I have with our pharmacist, which I just described. The second is that with PD, we changed drugs or dosage often. Sometimes the changes were due to negative reactions or side effects to a new drug, and other times the changes were just in dosage because the drug had to be titrated into use, beginning with a low dose, and ramping up over time. We don't know how our loved one will respond to new drugs until we try them. If we had been using a mail-order prescription service, that would have meant constant changes to the order, which could have meant many phone calls and even delays in receiving the correct medications.

There was a Parkinson's drug that my husband took for several years, and suddenly it was discontinued due to a manufacturing problem. That meant we had to wean him off this drug. Several years later it was on the market again, so we tried it a second time. It didn't seem as effective, so we discontinued it. Sometimes it seemed like his medications were changing every few months.

Also, since it is customary for drug companies to give doctors samples of new products, don't be afraid to ask for samples. They can be helpful for the first few days of trying a new medication, especially if they cause side effects and your loved one must stop taking the drug. The samples keep you from having to pay for drugs you can no longer use.

With Parkinson's disease, timing is everything in medications. The "go-to" drug to treat PD is Carbidopa/Levodopa (C/L), and it is only effective for a limited time, after which the patient may have "off" periods. That means it is important to take the next dose at exactly the correct time. Many people use a timer on the stove, a watch, or the computer to remind them of the next dose. The caregiver may need to help with medications when the patient can no longer manage this timing on their own. With a decline in cognition, they might eventually tend to forget or become confused regarding when the last dose of medication was taken, which would mean that they would take too much C/L or none. Both are problematic.

One more word of caution: Since medications can interact negatively with each other, it is very important that we share all information concerning every medication we take with every physician we see, no matter what their specialty is. This is when a printed list comes in handy. This list should include drugs purchased over the counter (OTC) and natural vitamin supplements, just to be safe.

Physicians

Your neurologist is the doctor that will see you through Parkinson's, so you need to have a good relationship with this doctor. We changed doctors several times near the beginning of our journey to find the right fit. Some neurologists specialize, so finding one that specializes in PD would be an advantage. However, you will need to find a doctor that fits your personalities as well, both yours and your loved one. It is important to be able to communicate easily and feel comfortable sharing personal information. You will need to trust your doctor's wisdom since they change medications and offer other suggestions.

Additionally, you will need to keep your specialists if you have other medical conditions, but you should alert EVERY doctor to the new diagnosis of Parkinson's disease. That will make a difference as they choose new medications and treatment going forward. It is important, above all, that you are open and honest with each of your doctors about your diagnosis and about what medications you take.

If you find a doctor who seems to turn a deaf ear to your loved one, that opens the door for you to advocate for them and make sure they are being heard. Don't be afraid to change doctors if you find that there is a problem with communication or compatibility. Having a good relationship with the front-office staff is also an advantage. When our favorite neurologist prescribed a very expensive drug for Carlton, we were thankful to the front-office staff for directing us to an online organization that helped make the drug affordable. They were also good to work with us on appointment times and medication refills.

Some people suggest that PD patients see a Movement Disorder Specialist (MDS) because PD affects mobility acutely. If it is possible, that is advisable. If not, don't worry. There are other options.

As soon as it is feasible, it is recommended that you attend doctors' appointments with your loved one. Even if they seem to be only mildly affected by PD at this time, there are several reasons to accompany them, especially to their neurology appointments. The most obvious reason is that one person may not be able to remember everything that the doctor says, but it is likely that two people will remember most of the pertinent information. As the disease progresses, having two people at each appointment will become even more critical. The neurologist will make suggestions to the caregiver about ways to make accommodations in the home to prevent falls, medications, and a myriad of other topics. This is the time when writing things down in a medical journal will help you remember them later. In addition, over the course of the disease, it is important that the neurologist know what type of support system your loved one has, and seeing YOU at appointments gives them insight into your level of care and commitment for the long term. That will help the doctor as they make decisions concerning your loved one's treatment and care.

When we, as caregivers, attend a doctor's appointment, we can help the doctor get a better perspective of our loved one's everyday life at home. For some reason, patients often allow a physician to only see them at their best. They walk better, talk better, and sit up straighter while in a neurologist's office. So, the caregiver can prompt their loved one to be sure to show how they act the other 99 percent of the time. The doctor needs to know the truth, but we might have to work hard to reveal it without demeaning our spouse. It is important to preserve their dignity while portraying a clear picture of their life at home.

Let me suggest that you schedule one virtual appointment with your neurologist. While this type of appointment is not preferred as the norm, having one tele-med visit could be eye-opening for your physician. We learned during the pandemic, in a tele-med doctor's visit, that seeing my husband in his own element and in his own home gave our neurologist new insight into his actual condition. I wish we had done this earlier because I believe it was informative for the doctor to see my husband more candidly.

Friends and Family

Even if this has not been true in the past, people are becoming very important for our loved one and the entire family. And those people fall into specific groups, none of which should be forgotten or overlooked. Each group will provide a specific type of support in our future. We can think of them like the petals of a flower.

The group closest to us, nearest to the center, might include both family and friends. These are the people that we hold most dear. These are the ones whom we will call on when we need emotional support throughout our journey. We need to keep them close. This means that when they say, "Please call me if you need anything," and we're pretty sure they mean it, we should make note of that. When the day comes that we really need help, and it probably will, we will know whom to call.

For us, this group included our two daughters, their husbands, and our seven grandchildren. My husband was formally diagnosed the year after our first two grandchildren were born, and they were followed by five more. That meant that all seven grandchildren grew up with a grandfather who had PD and was declining constantly. It was very natural and almost normal to see him decline, and the children began to notice it as they matured to a more observant age. It was just how "Papa" was.

That made it relatively easy to explain to them that Papa was getting worse, and that someday "soon" he would leave us and go to heaven. We talked about death with them openly, either when they asked a question, or when they hadn't seen him for several months and there had been a significant change. We treated death like any other topic—naturally.

Because they grew up around a handicapped person, I am proud to say that each of the children is comfortable in the presence of people with disabilities. They are usually quick to help someone in need, remembering how they helped their grandfather. To them, it is normal and natural to hold open the door, to pick up something that is dropped, or to push a wheelchair.

We also have a close group of friends who are always available, just as they were during the pandemic and Carlton's final days on this earth.

Other family members and friends who mean well but are not as always present in our lives are the next layer of petals of the flower, and they are still important. They provide another kind of support and encouragement. Even if they don't know much about our diagnosis, they are still a great resource for a chat when we need one. Sometimes it is refreshing to NOT talk about the illness, but just chat about what is happening in the rest of the world.

One of the best things we did early in our journey was finding a support group specifically for Parkinson's disease. We found ours quite by accident. A casual friend mentioned it because her friend was the leader of the group. Fifteen years later, I am so thankful for the friends and connections I made through that group. Their encouragement and support were invaluable. Search online for a group near you. In our group we shared successes by talking about medical equipment that was helpful, medication changes, physical therapy facilities, and many other topics that were specific to Parkinson's.

The bottom line is that certain people are crucial in that they provide encouragement, support, information, sharing of ideas, and physical help. At this time of diagnosis, we have no idea how long our PD journey will be. And the longer it lasts, the more we will need these people. So, let's hold our friends and family close, and work toward developing a relationship of trust and understanding with our physicians. These people will be the lifelines we will need to make this journey easier and more pleasant.

The first questions I asked after hearing the diagnosis were these: "How long does he have? How long do Parkinson's patients usually live?"

These are difficult questions to answer because each patient is unique, and no one can predict how long they will live with PD. In our support group we have known loved ones who lived six years, ten years, twenty-three years like my husband, and even twenty-six years and still functioned well. Some factors that contribute to length of life with PD are mentioned in this chapter such as pre-existing conditions, along with other conditions that your loved one develops, overall health, attitude, support system, family history, etc. The variables are nearly endless!

It is not healthy to dwell on "how much time we have left" nor what stage we are in. We can read about the stages of PD online, and that is helpful to some extent. But dwelling on it or obsessing over it is not in anyone's best interest. Instead, at this time of diagnosis, it is good to have the attitude that we will make the best of whatever time we have. This is the time to do the things we have always wanted to do, as we have means and ability.

Chapter Two
Living With It

Now that your loved one has Parkinson's, what do you do with it? The great news is that this first stage could last many years, so my best advice is to focus on living right now. Focus on how to get the most out of today, while preparing for tomorrow. Parkinson's may raise its ugly head from time to time, and you may have to deal with inconveniences due to it, but today is the day to live life to the fullest. As caregivers we can encourage our loved one to keep doing the things they love. This is the time to travel, write a book, enjoy hobbies old and new, and live life as normally as possible.

Adjusting Our Living Space

One of the first considerations is our home. If it is on more than one level, we might consider a move to a "ranch-style" home before mobility worsens. It is best to make changes like this before cognition becomes a problem also. If we wait, it is possible that our loved one will have difficulty adjusting to a new home due to confusion.

This is the time to make simple adjustments in our home. There are several accommodations we can easily make to keep our loved one from falling and make it easier for them to remain independent. It is wise to resist the urge to help them too soon because the longer they can care for themselves, the better. There may be a time when they cannot care for their basic needs so we will have to do it. But let's not rush that scenario.

When my husband was diagnosed with PD, we looked back over the last few years, and one thing we noticed was that nearly every time he stood up from a sitting position, he stumbled. Usually he commented, "Wow, the house moved. Did you feel it?" To which I would always answer in the negative. He was talking about his balance, the key to mobility, which is one of the huge issues with Parkinson's. For that reason, it is important to check your home for hazards that might cause your loved one to fall. As you walk through your home, shuffle your feet somewhat, which is what PD patients do, just to see if you catch your foot on anything. Common obstacles are throw rugs (the smaller ones are the most dangerous), piles of things they must navigate around (like books), or even small things that might be just out of their line of sight. Think of this exercise as preparing for a blind person visiting your home. Whatever you think might get in their way is something you can move to make your house safer for your loved one.

Often the furniture can be strategically placed, especially in a large room, to enable someone to hold onto the furniture as they walk throughout the house. The backs of tall chairs, the back of a couch, and sturdy furniture in the home are great for helping with balance.

It is expected that grab bars will need to be installed in the bathrooms. Take care to place them strategically to help in every area of that room. The next problem might be the tub or shower. We already had a walk-in shower with a very short lip, so we didn't have to make any other changes to our bathroom.

We have some dear friends who counseled us early in our PD journey that we should install ramps from the garage into the house, and from the back door of the house to the patio. There were only two to three steps involved in both places, and at the time I thought this was unnecessary. But when hubby began to need a walker and then a wheelchair, I was thankful for those ramps. It is difficult to see into the future, but we accepted a word from someone who had experience, and allowed them to install the ramps. We never regretted that decision.

They also encouraged us to put hand railings in our hallway. We have two hallways that intersect in a T, and we must use those passageways to get from the living space to the bedrooms. Our friends realized my husband would be walking that path several times a day.

So, we had beautiful handrails installed about three years after Hubby's diagnosis. Again, I didn't see that they were critical at that time. However, I cannot count the number of falls those railings have prevented. They have literally been lifesavers. Hubby did fall many times, but he was able to use the railings to pull himself back up.

If you have steps inside your house, even one step going into another room, consider putting caution tape along the edge of the step or painting the edge a different color. That will alert everyone that they are at the edge. Use this anywhere you want to draw attention to a change in pavement or flooring.

During our year at home due to COVID-19, we had one tele-med visit with our neurologist. At the opening of the Zoom session, he said, "Thank you for welcoming me into your home!" I was a bit shocked at that statement because I had not thought about the visual advantage of Zoom for him seeing our home. Then, after a few minutes of regular doctor visit-chatter, he said, "Please take me on a tour of your home. I'd like to see where your husband sleeps and the bathroom he uses."

That caused me to be quite uncomfortable. I had not planned on this. My next thought was, *I hope I made his bed this morning!* So, I left Hubby in his chair and took my phone and the doctor on a walking tour through the house. As I walked, the doctor said, "Show me the floor." We have wood floors with no rugs in that area because that made walking easier for Hubby. So, I aimed the phone at the floor to show him. He said, "Very good. No rugs." He also commented on the fact that there were no piles of clutter or decorative things that might get in Hubby's way. In my mind I was saying, *Whew! I passed that test!*

Then I got to Hubby's bedroom. He had a hospital bed, but in our eight to ten years with this doctor, I'm not sure he had ever asked about that. I showed him the bed (already made, thankfully), and he commented on the fact that it was a hospital bed. He asked if Hubby was overall comfortable while sleeping. I answered in the affirmative.

After that I walked to the bathroom. We had already installed grab bars near the toilet and shower, and then in the shower itself. He commented on those as well, noting how important they are to prevent falling.

When reflecting later about this tele-med call, I believe all neurologists could benefit from such a call. However, I believe it should be done earlier in the journey of Parkinson's. Seeing the home situation would help the doctor understand the environment in which their patient lives. It would also help the family understand some of the seemingly small things they can do to make their home safer and prevent falls and subsequent injuries.

I am so thankful for the little things we did early after Carlton's diagnosis, like installing the railings in the hallway and the grab bars in the bathrooms. And as PD progressed, we had to keep adjusting. When there was a new development, we worked to find a new equilibrium. We sometimes struggled to find that new balance, but eventually we achieved a new normal.

It may not be found in many books on the subject, but we discovered a rule of thumb about Parkinson's patients: They can only focus on one thing at a time, especially as the disease progresses. Eventually this truth affec`ts every area of life, such as driving, working outside the home, and staying home alone.

For us, driving took care of itself about five years into his diagnosis. We have other friends who are still driving at twenty years into Parkinson's. So, there is no rule to follow regarding how long they can drive safely. Several issues are at stake when making this decision: their response time when faced with a sudden situation that requires immediate action, their anxiety while driving, their eyesight, and their ability to multitask. All drivers must be able to respond quickly enough to get out of the way of approaching traffic, foreign objects, or pedestrians that come into their path. And while responding, they must also think about the cars in adjacent lanes, their speed, etc. When my husband realized he could not turn the wheel quickly enough to get out of the way of other cars, he became concerned and readily gave up driving. If your loved one is resistant about giving up driving, you may need to get creative, or you might ask for the help of a loved one or physician to convince them of the wisdom of giving up their keys.

Working outside the home was a bit tricky, but he also gave that up voluntarily. At the time of his diagnosis, Carlton was employed by a large company as a project manager. He had a small office where he worked alone much of the day, but when he met with his team, he had to move to a large conference room. This meant that he often had to walk down the hallway to a meeting room while carrying his drink and laptop, one in each hand. At first that wasn't a problem, even though his steps were slow. Over time, however, he began to shuffle his feet and felt unsteady, so he left the drink at his desk to have one hand free to balance himself against the wall if he stumbled.

Eventually he had to leave the laptop back at his desk and use both hands to stabilize himself for fear of falling on his way to the conference room. He had reached the point where he could literally only concentrate on one thing at a time—walking. He realized his workdays were numbered. He was coming to the end of his ability to work outside of our home. (This was pre-COVID and working at home was less popular and not as accessible.)

But his company did allow him to work two days a week from home for a while. However, that lasted only a few months. They needed someone onsite, so he retired about eight years after his diagnosis on long-term disability.

Thankfully, Carlton stayed home alone for the next ten years while I worked. In the next chapter I will explain how we knew it was time to hire a sitter for him.

Exercise

Both patient and caregiver need to exercise as much as possible by doing physical activities that are enjoyable. We count every activity that gets us moving as exercise. The longer we can exercise, the longer we can move because staying active now is the key to staying active longer.

During the first few years after my husband was diagnosed with PD, he walked a half-mile every day to get to his job because the city bus route stopped a quarter-mile from his building, so he walked the rest of the way twice each day. I believe this helped him stay mobile longer.

In that instance we did not call it "exercise," so he did not dread walking. It was just part of getting to his job. So, if your spouse is already active, congratulate them and encourage them to keep going.

If they are not really moving much, or if you feel more exercise is needed, great options are available. Many programs are offered at gyms, senior centers, YMCAs, or other meeting places. They range from free to expensive, and grueling hard work to fun! Some are designed to be done while standing, but chair exercise is another alternative, especially when balance is a problem.

One of the best programs to keep your loved one moving and energized is the **"Big and Loud"** program. Many who have gone through this program have been helped by it, especially when they continue those exercises at home. One advantage of this program is that it addresses both speaking and moving. Another benefit is that it can be done whether the participants are newly diagnosed or in the late stages of any disease.

Another program, **"Move and Shout"** (perhaps a take-off on the **"Big and Loud"**), was recommended by a speech therapist we met. She suggested that we do this together, and that turned out to be a great plan. It gave us something "active" to do as a couple. We made it part of a regular routine for a while by using videos online. We competed, as we did in many areas, which made it fun for both of us.

Recently I read about the British Gymnastics Foundation, which has published videos of exercises for seniors. "The programme is chair-based and helps to improve memory, balance, flexibility and co-ordination." It is also free and online, and it can be done in groups or pairs. This one is called **"Love to Move."**

If motivation is an obstacle with your loved one, you might consider spinning this idea of exercise as if YOU are the one needing it, not them. You can say that they would be doing you a huge favor if they would do it with you since you need some prodding. A little bit of "carrot and stick" might also work.

Truthfully, any kind of movement is valuable, especially as the disease progresses, so we cannot give up. We must keep trying different things that might help keep our loved one moving, even a little.

One of the pitfalls of having a degenerative disease is falling into the trap of apathy. We see this often in Parkinson's patients, and it can occur at any time—immediately after diagnosis (thinking it is the end of one's life), or when movement becomes difficult. As caregivers sometimes it seems as if we are constantly building up our loved one emotionally to keep them from becoming apathetic or giving up.

The goal for all of us is to stay positive. Our loved one can still do many of the things they previously enjoyed, even if they must do them slower or on a smaller scale than previously. So, keep at this. With PD, the major enemy is apathy. Once apathy sets in, usually one's health will decline. Maintaining a positive attitude and moving often means your loved one will be able to move longer on this journey.

MEDICAL EQUIPMENT

Along this journey, your family will probably accumulate several types of medical equipment. We all want to keep our loved one walking as long as possible to preserve their independence and keep them active. But after removing all physical hazards in the home to prevent falls, if falling is still a problem, we can add simple devices to keep them safe.

The symptoms our loved one exhibits will dictate when and if each piece of equipment is necessary. For instance, when he/she has trouble walking and stumbles or falls often, the doctor may suggest a cane or a walker, and eventually a wheelchair. Medicare will pay for some of these aids with a prescription from the doctor. Be sure to ask if you are eligible for that.

The easiest addition might be a **cane**. There are some decorative canes available for purchase that can even become a conversation piece, or you can decorate or paint your own if desired. My husband bought his first one online, and when it arrived it was too tall (long), so he had to saw it off to shorten it to fit him. Later, people gave him other types of canes, but the first one was his favorite.

We bought our first **walker** because we wanted the type with a seat and compartment for storage underneath it. Medicare paid for a standard walker, which was more convenient because it was lighter, and acquiring another one meant we could keep them in different parts of the house. There is no timetable for how long our loved one should use any of these devices because it's different for everyone. The goal is to keep our loved one from falling, so we should encourage the use of whatever it takes to keep them safe.

During his experience with Parkinson's, my husband had several **wheelchairs.** Some were gifts from friends, and they were very much appreciated. We discovered that even when Hubby could walk comfortably at home using only a cane, we had to resort to a wheelchair in public. Since public distances are so much greater than distances in the home, he was tiring too quickly, even just walking from the car to the door of a store.

Medicare paid for a well-equipped wheelchair after we got a prescription from our neurologist. The doctor was very specific regarding the official prescription because he wanted to make certain it had specific features. In addition, we bought a "transport" chair to have a lighter option and a smaller one that fit better through the doorways of our home. The transport chair was also easier to lift into the car.

Our neurologist was knowledgeable about which devices were necessary and which ones were covered under Medicare. We also talked with other patients in our Parkinson's support group to find out which devices worked for them.

In general, we found that people were very courteous to us when Hubby was using a walker or sitting in a wheelchair. That signaled to them that he had a physical disability, so strangers would hold the door or give us the opportunity to go first through a door. Without any medical equipment, they could not easily tell that he was disabled.

Another big purchase was his **lift chair**. When my husband could not get up from the chair without help, we knew it was time for that type of recliner chair. Our first one was handed down from a friend. But that one was well used, so it didn't last long. However, it showed us how invaluable the lift feature was.

The largest piece of medical equipment we acquired was the **hospital bed**. My husband was in the hospital to have his gall bladder removed, and before we left the hospital, they assigned him home healthcare assistance. When they came to the house, they noticed the trouble he had getting out of bed, so they ordered a hospital bed provided by Medicare. The height of the bed was adjustable, and in those early days he could adjust it himself by pushing a button. He even liked the head raised slightly to help with his sleep apnea.

Remember that there is no set timetable for the use of these devices. You may acquire some before you actually need them, which is perfectly acceptable. If you wonder if it is the right time to get a particular device, just do it. The comfort and convenience for you and your loved one are the goals in all of this. Your doctor and other people may not understand, but you are caring for your loved one every day, and you know what is needed. There is no wrong or right order to do this.

SYMPTOMS AND SIDE EFFECTS

The symptoms that propelled your loved one to the doctor originally to seek a diagnosis may be very different than the ones that drove my husband to do the same thing. Parkinson's can affect every system of the body one way or another, and it seems to do that in no specific order. Also, while some symptoms last throughout the entire journey, others are just a temporary nuisance. Over the course of his twenty-three-year journey, Carlton had difficulty with each of these issues at one time or another. But not all PD patients experience every one of these symptoms:

- Mobility issues such as shuffling, freezing, falling, and festination
- Leaning
- Sleeping
- Eating
- Smells
- Speech
- Double vision/dry eyes
- Dental health/dry mouth
- Constipation/Diarrhea
- Choking
- Anxiety/panic/depression
- Dysgraphia (tiny handwriting)
- Both high and low blood pressure

Those are the major problems associated with Parkinson's, but some others are found quite often: apathy, stiffness, skin problems (extremely dry or oily skin), general overall pain, sweating, drooling, incontinence, and sexual problems. While these are not specifically addressed here, they can be annoying at best and problematic at worst. The internet has suggestions for mitigating each of them, should they occur. And if they persist, we should consult our physician.

You may be asking the first question WE asked when confronted with one of these, "Are all of these related to PD?"

The answer is, "Yes, they can be."

The next question might be, "Are they always?"

And the answer is, "No, but they can be."

Researchers and physicians do not agree on the cause for many of these symptoms. Their explanations include general symptoms of PD, side effects of medication typical for long-term PD, aging, and the results of drugs taken for other conditions.

In the long run, it doesn't always matter why one has any of these problems. Our physician is usually focused on the cause, but we must address the effects. They are still problems, whether we know their source or not, and at home we must find solutions or make accommodations. We have to live with them!

Some problems can be solved or overcome. (That was true for Carlton's experience with dry eyes.) Some are present for a time, and then they quietly go away. (That was true for change of smell and taste with my husband.) Others will be with us for the duration, so we learn to live with them. (For us, that was the "leaning.") These can best be described as inconveniences. So, perhaps we can consider each symptom as minor until they become major!

It helps to make notes on the ways we treated each symptom or solved the problems in case they come back. The problems that remain will need to be managed or handled. How can we adjust our lives, homes, or schedules to accommodate this new normal? Let's discuss them one at a time.

Mobility Solutions

Problems with mobility vary as with other symptoms, but they will likely progress and not fade away. The goal is to keep our loved one as mobile as possible for as long as possible. Several different kinds of problems with walking typically plague PD patients—freezing, festination, shuffling, stumbling, and falling.

Shuffling and stumbling are usually among the first signs of PD. We noticed both of these before Carlton was ever diagnosed. I will confess that I said to him often, "Honey, pick up your feet! You are shuffling." He just couldn't, but I did not understand that yet.

Freezing is common in many PD patients. By freezing we mean that the brain just refuses to pass on information to the rest of the body, so the feet just stop. They cannot move, even though the brain is trying to tell them to move. This can happen anywhere, but for us it usually happened when Hubby approached a doorway. When he was still walking, even with a cane, if we were entering a public building like a restaurant, we would reach the doorway, and he would stop. He just froze. He could not move. And if other customers wanted to go through that same doorway at the same time, it became awkward. It was as if they all wanted to say, "Go on through. Why are you stopping? Let's get going!" But there was nothing I could do or say to get him to move on through the doorway. (Yes, a few times I said, "Honey, just go through the doorway!" But again, it did no good.) He just froze. In his mind he was trying to get his feet to move, but his feet were not receiving the message from his brain. Thankfully, we never had a stranger yell at him or become frustrated by his inability to move. Somehow, they seemed to understand that he just couldn't move. The cane or walker he was using signaled to them that he was having difficulty. Most people were very patient.

That is Parkinson's at its best—or worst. Freezing happens when you least expect it or want it to happen. (Parkinson's involves a lack of dopamine in the brain, which causes the brain to short-circuit so that it cannot relay messages from one part to another. So, in these moments of freezing, the brain is telling the feet to move, but the feet are not responding.)

Throughout our PD journey, we used several different physical therapists at different times. It was interesting to hear each one of them give a different suggestion regarding cues I could give hubby to help him "unfreeze" while walking. Here are some of our favorite tips: *counting* (which made him think he was marching), *using masking tape* on the floor to give him a mark to aim for (this made the floor look like it had a pattern for him to follow), and *singing*. Each of these worked sometimes, but none worked every time. We used the masking tape at home down our hallway, and it was very successful—until it wasn't. Of course, this was not something we could do in public.

However, we realized quickly that if Hubby was in the wheelchair, freezing was not a problem. And usually, a stranger was quick to hold the door open for me to push the wheelchair through. That saved us from the embarrassment of him freezing.

Another difficulty while walking is **festination**. Festination means "the shortening of each step in a long gait sequence, together with an increase in gait speed and involuntary forward-leaning of the trunk." In laymen's terms, it occurs when your loved one takes shorter and shorter steps, which causes them to lean forward and eventually topple over face first. This is typical with PD patients.

This mostly occurs because the patient walks on the front or ball of the foot, which causes them to take smaller and smaller steps, which, in turn, causes them to lean forward, making them think they are falling. And many times, they DO fall.

In the middle stages of Parkinson's, the weakening of the body core can also cause leaning. This is sometimes called the Pisa Syndrome. My husband leaned to the right. He first noticed it while sitting on the bed because there were no arm rests like the arms on the chair. And after sitting in a wing back chair or recliner, it was obvious that his core was so weak he could not keep himself sitting upright without the arms of the chair.

Even in his lift chair, he always leaned to the right. We put a pillow beside him to keep him straight. But when the leaning got worse, his CNA told us about a wedge we could buy to keep him from falling over. That was a huge help.

Sleeping

At every visit our neurologist asked us about sleep patterns. "Is he sleeping more, less, or about the same? Is he having difficulty falling asleep or staying asleep?" The bottom line is that PD can cause changes in sleep patterns, and it seems to do this randomly.

When Carlton was first put on Carbidopa/Levodopa (C/L), he slept constantly. I would have to wake him to eat. And almost every time the dosage of C/L was changed, his sleep pattern also changed. There was a period of about five years when he needed a sleeping pill to help him fall asleep. This was a controlled substance, so we worried about him becoming addicted to it. But with a degenerative disease, that was not something we needed to stress about. After a few years, it seemed like suddenly he didn't need that pill. Knowing Carlton the way I did, I believe he had to learn to turn off his brain so he could sleep. He needed that medication to accomplish that for a while, but there came a time when PD had affected his brain to the point that he did not need medication to relax his brain. At least that is how it seemed to me.

It is true that PD affects sleep and the brain is constantly changing due to the degenerative nature of PD. So, it stands to reason that our loved one's sleep patterns might change as the disease progresses.

Eating and Dental Health

It is important to pay attention to dental health during Parkinson's, especially regarding sharing your PD diagnosis with your dentist. There are several things that may happen in the mouth of a PD patient. The teeth may shift spatially, which will affect chewing. If the bite lined up previously, as PD progresses, the bite may change.

The ability for our loved one to hold open their mouth will lessen over time, so preventative care becomes the best course of action. The first thing our dentist recommended was an electric toothbrush. Hubby could not move his hand back and forth to move a regular toothbrush, so the new toothbrush was a huge help. He also suggested mouthwash for problems with dry mouth. Thankfully, this symptom finally went away. Consistent dental care will aid in keeping the mouth healthy and free of infection.

Swallowing will likely become more difficult and taking pills can become a problem—and we will be taking a LOT of pills! In our experience, taking pills in applesauce was the best way to swallow the many pills needed to keep moving with PD. We opened capsules or used a mortar and pestle to crush pills, and then we sprinkled the contents into a spoonful of applesauce for ease in swallowing.

Carlton had a good appetite until the final three to six months of his life. We were thankful for that, but there was one short period of time when nothing tasted good. We attributed that to a new medication he was taking. He said everything tasted metallic, and while I was cooking his favorite foods, he would step outside because he said the smell was sickening! This lasted only a short time, and gradually his taste and smell returned to "normal." We have heard this is typical with many patients, but it lasts longer for some.

During my husband's journey, he had three different swallowing tests performed by different speech therapists. Each one was extremely beneficial. The first one showed a tendency toward aspiration of liquid and even of solid food, such as a cracker. She warned us of this and gave us advice about which foods to avoid. She also mentioned maintaining good dental health.

Each speech therapist also gave my husband tips about speaking louder and more clearly. There are several different programs that help PD patients with movement and speech. One such program is **"BIG AND LOUD."** This is an excellent way to keep moving and improve communication and interaction. When attending a session is not possible, something similar is available online.

Soft speech is a huge problem for PD patients. Sometimes it is one of the first signs that one has PD. And for some, it just gets worse and worse over the years until they can barely be heard at the end of their life. That is how it was with my husband. Each speech therapist gave him good hints about how to strengthen his voice and keep his volume loud enough to be heard. But it still got harder and harder for him to keep up the volume. It is not enough for us as caregivers to say, "Speak louder!" because they cannot, at least not for long periods of time and not consistently. Their singular focus means they can concentrate on only one thing at a time—saying the correct words that make sense or speaking/yelling loudly. They cannot do both at the same time.

Eye Health

It is equally important to not neglect eye health when you have PD. Some optometrists will tell you that PD does not affect the eyes. However, as we observe our loved one on this PD journey, and as we watch a weakening of the core muscles, it is not a stretch to believe that the muscles in the eyes will weaken as well. Hubby began seeing double in about the tenth year of his disease. His optometrist originally said there was no correlation. But we have since seen double vision listed in several online documents that include symptoms or side effects of PD. It is also listed as common on the **Michael J. Fox website.**

There was also a period where hubby had dry eyes, which could stem from the fact that PD patients sometimes do not close their eyes completely when they sleep, and while awake, sometimes they blink less than usual. That meant that his eyes were always open, so they dried out easily. Our optometrist recommended eye drops that helped with this, but the condition lasted two-plus years.

Bathroom Problems

With decreased mobility and dexterity, it is normal for our loved one to need help in the bathroom one day. As with every other area in the house, we want them to remain independent as long as possible, so there are devices to help in this room as well.

Consider a raised toilet seat, a bidet, a roll-in shower stall, a shower chair, a hand-held shower sprayer, a power toothbrush, a Waterpic®, etc. Those are the first steps for accommodations in the bathroom. Hopefully, they will be enough to last a very long time.

With Parkinson's disease, there is also the constant swing between constipation and diarrhea. For many years, it seemed as if we never found a happy medium. It was always one extreme or the other. This problem causes untold difficulties for PD patients. To help with this, we first consulted our primary care doctor. When her suggestions didn't help, we researched online, yet our most effective treatment/solution came from other PD caregivers.

As caregivers, we must decide how extreme we will allow the situation to become before consulting our primary care physician. On one occasion I took my husband to the emergency room on day ten of constipation because he was very uncomfortable. That was after I had tried every possible home remedy. It took an extreme enema to relieve the problem, and the hospital staff told me there was no way I could ever have done that at home.

We experienced this problem for about eight years, but it stopped after he had his gall bladder removed. This was not an expected outcome of the surgery, but we were very thankful.

Relationships

During our time with PD, I noticed that our relationship changed from being husband and wife partners to being patient and caregiver. This may seem obvious to the outsider, but when it is occurring personally, it is earth-shaking. If the patient and caregiver were quite compatible and comfortable with each other while sharing responsibilities and decision-making in the marriage/home, it is likely that the relationship will change as PD progresses. It can feel as if we are losing our best friend. Our loved one may seem to be pulling away emotionally while they are becoming less mobile and more dependent.

One of the most telling aspects for us regarded finances. When first diagnosed, Hubby was totally handling the finances of our family. The progression, without reference to timing, went something like this:

First: Hubby couldn't write the checks. His handwriting became illegible (dysgraphia). So, he asked me to sit with him as he entered the data into the spreadsheet on the computer, and then he told me how to make out each check.

Second: Hubby couldn't make the mouse for the computer work easily. So, he asked me to sit beside him at the computer while I entered the data into the spreadsheet he was using.

Third: He sat beside me and watched television while I filled out the spreadsheet and paid the bills. But he was there in case I had questions.

The rest of this story is in the next chapter. But it is easy to see that there is a gradual transfer taking place. It is normal and natural, and felt organic and comfortable. Looking back, I can see that we were becoming patient and caregiver. Our relationship was shifting.

Medications

The "go-to" medication for Parkinson's disease is carbidopa/levodopa, which comes in different forms. It is normal for caregivers to ask other caregivers about the dosage their spouse is taking; however, we must be careful to not fall into the trap of thinking that all Parkinson's patients should be taking the same amount or type of C/L. It might be best to ask our neurologist if we have questions about that.

First, it is of utmost importance that Parkinson's meds be taken on time. Their effectiveness is timed, and when that runs out, it is almost as if someone turned the switch to "off." The window of the viability of the popular PD drug, Carbidopa/Levodopa (C/L), is narrow, and it changes as the disease progresses. Every time we notice that our loved one's meds wear off before the time to take the next dose, we need to inform the doctor so they can change the dosage or timing. This may happen often immediately after diagnosis as the doctor gauges your loved one's response to the C/L. Then it will likely settle for a while when it feels as if you are on a plateau. Suddenly things will change, which will indicate a need for a change in dosage. Don't be alarmed at this.

One more thing about timing. (This is foreign to many staff members in the hospital.) This means that if your loved one must go to the hospital, be sure to notify your neurologist. Also, take some extra C/L with you in case the hospital pharmacy cannot provide that particular medication, or the staff doesn't share your feelings about the need to give your loved one their medications at a particular time. You will need to advocate for this. (There is more to explain about taking our loved one to the hospital in the next chapter.)

Since the timing of taking C/L is everything, when we notice that our loved one cannot remember when they took their last dose or how many pills they took, or our loved one shows cognitive decline, it may be time for us to take over the administering of medications. This will allow us to be sure they are taking the right dose at the right time, and it keeps us from worrying about it.

It is not common to think of pain as a symptom of Parkinson's disease. However, it is listed on the Michael J. Fox website because many PD patients do experience chronic general pain. Whatever the source of the pain, now is the time to get them into a pain management regimen so the pain does not take over their entire life and future.

There also could be anxiety and frustration that accompany Parkinson's. Patients become anxious when they freeze and cannot move. They become frustrated because they cannot do the things they used to do. The good news is that this anxiety and frustration can be minimized with medication. The flip side is that many of our loved ones do not want to add "one more pill," so they refuse to talk with their doctor about those symptoms. They may deny that they feel those emotions, but we who see them at home have evidence to the contrary.

As caregivers we can sometimes arrange to speak with the doctor privately to inform them that our loved one is having difficulty in this area. This might help open a conversation that will lead to a solution to the problem. (One way I did this was by leaving my husband in the examining room, saying that I was going to the restroom. While out of the room, I spoke to the nurse about my concerns.)

Depression

When Carlton was first diagnosed, he mentioned to the doctor that he had difficulty with depression in the past, even though he had never been medicated for it. Thankfully, his neurologist gave him a small dose of anti-anxiety medication. That made a huge improvement in his attitude, and I credit those drugs with helping him have a positive outlook about Parkinson's disease.

After about ten years, however, he noticed those old feelings coming back, so he spoke with his neurologist again. This prompted the doctor to give him a heavier dosage of the same drug he had been taking, and that restored his positive attitude. Again, I am thankful that his doctor listened to him and gave him the medication he needed.

When thinking of Parkinson's from the patient's perspective, we can only imagine how it must feel to realize that you are losing ground. When we understand the degenerative nature of PD, it helps us understand how our loved one must feel.

Family and Friends

Family and friends are important in this stage as well. This is the time to welcome visits while our loved one can still communicate and enjoy them. Having positive interaction with friends and family will give us hope for the future and dispel apathy. We do not know how much of a cognitive decline is ahead, so we must seize the day!

CHAPTER THREE
Advanced Parkinson's Disease

Our loved one did not ask for Parkinson's, and neither did we ask to be a caregiver. When the disease is newly diagnosed and in the early stages, both the caregiver and loved one are moving through uncharted territory, still in a partnership. In some ways we can keep an attitude of adventure as we tackle some of the hurdles of Parkinson's disease together.

However, as our loved one becomes less able to help overcome the difficulties of this disease, we become the primary persons attempting to scale the mountain, pulling them up with us as we go. We have entered the next season where we become the ones having to navigate life while carrying them on our back, so to speak. None of this is news to you if you are a caregiver. You are probably already feeling the strain.

GETTING HELP

But we are not totally alone. It is becoming increasingly necessary to call on our close family, dearest friends, and faith community to help us through the next phase of this journey. There is hope, my caregiver friend, and we do not have to navigate these uncharted waters alone. Others have gone before us, and we should not hesitate to ask for their support in whatever area we need it.

Since we cannot neglect our own health and well-being, we might need to ask for help from others to give us respite or relief from time to time. In general, if people have offered to help, they will be happy to sit with our loved one while we go out. At first, we will only need casual assistance. But as the necessary care becomes more medical in nature, we may need to find other resources to find qualified medical professionals to stay with our loved one. There are many resources to help with this, and local support groups are a great place to begin. The VA offers help if we qualify, and social services in our area might also be a good resource. When we need help, we need to keep looking until we find it. Our physical and mental health are important!

SELF-CARE

Sometimes we focus so much on caring for our loved ones that we forget to take care of ourselves. This is normal but not advisable. Also, since this is a marathon of a journey, we don't know how long we will be providing caregiving. We will need personal strength and endurance to finish the task.

When people mention self-care, they are implying that we must take care of our own bodies, minds, emotions, and spirits. The following are some brief suggestions for each one.

Physically we need to stay active. One way to track our activity would be to purchase a wearable device like an Apple Watch. It reminds us when to stand, counts how many steps we've taken in a day, and measures our heart rate both while active and at rest. It is imperative that we care for ourselves physically during each stage of our loved one's illness. In the first few stages we can go out to an exercise class and make regular check-ups with our doctor. However, in the advanced stage(s) it becomes harder to leave them, so we may need to opt for Zoom classes or online videos for exercises. Nevertheless, we cannot ignore our own health.

Mentally we need to stay active also. Some of us read, some work puzzles, some make craft items, and some like to write. As you think about exercising your mind, what do you do to keep it active? Would you like to learn to do something new and different, such as learning another language, making some type of craft, or cooking something new in the kitchen? Learning keeps the mind active, and that is our goal.

Emotional wellness can come from several avenues. When our loved one becomes distant emotionally, we must look to others to fill that need for emotional support and affirmation. We have talked about the importance of close friends and family to help us care for our loved one with Parkinson's, but they are also important for our own personal well-being. Sometimes we just need to vent our frustrations, talk about something else to get our mind off caregiving, or perhaps we just need to hear someone tell us we're doing a good job. Our inner circle of friends and family can provide that emotional support.

It is entirely possible that many friends and family will ask about our loved one, the patient, but they may never ask how WE are doing. We need to lean in toward those who ask about us, the ones who consider our needs. They are our inner circle who provide our emotional support.

Spiritual wellness is crucial to our overall health. We can begin with meditation or prayer since both quiet the soul and mind. By centering ourselves, we can attain spiritual balance and recharge our emotional and spiritual batteries. The next step involves community. It is healthy to communicate on a spiritual level with like-minded people as well as those who have different perspectives to challenge us. We are spiritual creatures who gravitate toward the Source of life greater than ourselves. This takes our focus from ourselves and our situation, which can become all-consuming, and creates an attitude of thankfulness for our many blessings, giving us hope.

From experience I can tell you that we need to care for our own selves as caregivers. Self-care keeps us mentally, physically, emotionally, and spiritually healthy, and it is up to us to attend to it. When our loved one passes from this life, we will still have more life to live, and if we want to enjoy it, we must care for our own bodies and minds now.

In this advanced stage of Parkinson's, various symptoms can become more problematic. Here are some suggestions about how to cope with them.

Mobility

For Parkinson's patients, mobility becomes a huge problem as the disease progresses. It sometimes occurs that in the final stage of PD, the patient will be unable to walk—first confined to a wheelchair, and then perhaps eventually confined to a bed because he/she cannot stand or even sit up on their own. Thankfully, there are various resources to aid in caring for people in these circumstances. Medical professionals, especially certified nursing assistants (CNAs), are a great resource to help when that time comes. Those who are experienced have seen other patients with similar problems and have also seen workable solutions. Our experience with CNAs from hospice companies is that if they did not already know the solution to a problem, they would ask their colleagues to find the best solution to keep my husband comfortable because that is their goal.

At the end of this chapter there is a lengthy section on the pros and cons of hospice, with a description of our experience with them.

Bathroom Problems

In the previous chapter I mentioned constipation versus diarrhea, and I explained that Hubby would swing from one to the other, regardless of any precautions we took. We tried the natural remedies, and then when his constipation became worse, we tried enemas and suppositories. It is advisable to talk with your primary care doctor and neurologist about this so they can avoid prescribing any medications that may have side effects that could be causing either of these conditions.

My final word on bathroom problems concerns catheters and incontinence. In later stages of PD, it is important for us as caregivers to communicate with ALL of our loved ones' doctors, including their urologist (or gynecologist). Each doctor must know of every problem at home to advise us on the best way to keep them safe and comfortable at the end of their life. At a regular visit with my hubby's urologist, I mentioned that he was falling every time he got up to go to the bathroom. That meant he was falling three to four times a day, or any time I could not be there to help him. After trying other things, the doctor decided that a Foley catheter was the best solution to the problem. He actually said to us, "I was thinking it was about time for this." This helped tremendously, but it was not without issues itself. In the long run it was the best solution for Carlton for the final eighteen months of his life.

Every patient is different, which means that not everyone with PD will become incontinent, but there are products available to help if they do. Medical professionals can inform us about options if we are open and honest about the behavior of our loved one at home. Embarrassment needs to be placed in the past at this point. Our loved one's safety and comfort is the primary goal.

Eating

Carlton had a great appetite until the last few months of his life, especially for sweets. This seems to be true of many PD patients. (While sweets may not be the healthiest thing for them to eat at this stage of life, healthy eating is not the main goal. So, perhaps we could give in to their wishes to keep peace and allow them things that give them joy.)

There came a time when he started coughing every time he ate. I anticipated this because of literature I had read, so I changed our diet slightly, eliminating meat and chewy foods. That helped for a while, but eventually he could not chew at all, so we moved to mashed potatoes, mashed cauliflower, and mashed "anything else I could think of." I added chicken gravy or beef gravy on top to give him a little protein and flavor. At this point we were deep into experimenting with foods, never knowing from meal to meal what he could eat without coughing or choking. Aspiration pneumonia was our biggest worry. He also began to panic every time he choked, thinking he might get something lodged in his throat and not be able to breathe. The nutritional value of the food was obviously not a high priority at this point.

He also began to have a lot of phlegm in his throat in the last month. Our CNA and hospice nurse showed me how to use a suction machine to give him relief from that periodically. Eventually we had to use it several times a day.

Eye Health

In the later stage of his disease, my husband also had problems with the light from the computer, double vision, and even loss of vision. We are not convinced that all of these were a result of Parkinson's, but they were bothersome, nonetheless. We took him to a low-vision clinic in our town at the suggestion of his optometrist, where they gave us some great practical hints to help his vision. They also had a gift shop where we found several items to keep him safe and independent at home, items designed to help people with poor eyesight.

Hospitals

As Parkinson's progresses, it is advisable to avoid hospitals whenever possible. As our loved one's cognition declines, so does their ability to adapt to new environments. And the hospital is definitely a new environment with new people, new rules, new smells, new routines, and new foods. One of the first problems we encounter is that we are experts on the care of our loved ones, and the hospital staff is not. They do not know our routine, which is sacred to us.

We live our lives on a time schedule, and because C/L must be taken on time to be effective, we understand what happens when it is not taken on time. Hospital employees don't usually think that way. If you tell them you take C/L three times a day, they will give it to you sometime in the morning, sometime around midday, and sometime in the evening. Even if you specify that you take it at 8:00 a.m., then at noon, then at 4:00 p.m., it is not likely that you will receive it at those times.

And then there is the problem of C/L itself. Hospitals like to provide you with the medications you take while there, but if you take the time-released version of C/L, they may not have it, especially in the dosage you are accustomed to. It is wise to take your prescription medications with you in their original bottles if you must go to the hospital. You may not need them, but it will save you a trip back home if you DO find it necessary to use your own.

My husband was in the hospital only twice during his last years of life. The first time was the extreme constipation event. During that two-day stay, they discovered that his potassium was extremely low, so they gave him massive amounts through his IV. For most people, this time in the hospital should not have caused any problems, but Carlton quickly became disoriented and confused. Suddenly, he became immobile and overwhelmed with being in a new place. The staff constantly asked me if he was like this at home, just a day ago, to which I replied, "No! I cannot imagine why he is like this here." As it was, when we pulled into the garage at home, he asked, "Whose house is this?" My heart sank, and I wondered if he would ever recover from this loss of memory and cognition. Thankfully he did, but it took about a month.

His last trip to the hospital was eighteen months before he passed, and the cognitive decline was even worse this time. It only took three hours in the emergency room for his physical and mental condition to decline to a place that was lower than it had ever been. This time we made sure he was never alone since he could no longer make himself heard or understood. During this hospital stay they removed his gall bladder under general anesthetic. Following the surgery, he could not stand alone, and his cognition was even less.

As a result of his confusion and decline, the social worker did not want him to be released to me. Instead, she wanted him to go to a rehab facility. That was a shock to me, but I never relayed that message to him. After talking with my daughters and a trusted medical professional who knew him well, it was decided that we would bring him home. My thought was that if he had to go to one more strange place, his mind would not be able to handle it, and he would decline even faster. When he came home three days later, the medical staff offered the suggestion of hospice, both for his sake and mine because I could not take care of him alone.

Since that time, I have talked with many other caregivers who have experienced similar reactions from their loved ones, both to the new environment of a hospital and the administration of a general anesthetic. So, when given a choice, I would choose an alternative to the hospital.

Anticipatory Grief

The grief that we feel before our loved one passes is called "anticipatory grief," and it is painful. It is also helpful because we process the transitioning better, for the most part. During this stage of PD, we are already seeing a decline in our loved one, and we realize that we must treasure each day. We are beginning the process of grieving while they are with us. This is normal, natural, and to be expected. When we channel these emotions in a positive way, it makes us thankful for Parkinson's disease and the time we have with our loved one. We have time to reminisce over memories, time to apologize if need be, time to enjoy life together a while longer, and time to prepare for their passing into the next life. The gift of time is a true blessing. It is up to us to use it wisely.

During this final stage, many of us feel the gap widening between ourselves and our loved one with Parkinson's. Here is the rest of the story about how we handled our finances. In the previous chapter I described the first three stages of how I began to take over the spreadsheet and our checkbook.

Step four involved Carlton staying in his lift chair in the family room while I went to the computer to keep up with the finances. I could still go out to where he was seated to ask questions, and when I was finished, he asked me how much money we had left.

Step five occurred organically. I barely noticed it was happening until one day I realized we had passed into a new era. Carlton didn't ask anything about our money. He didn't ask if I had paid the bills, something he had always asked previously. He didn't ask how much money we had left, another traditional question. We had entered the period where it took all his energy and brain power to just stay alive. There was not room for any other issues. He also stopped asking about our daughters and their families, something that was previously his habit.

It is as if they are pulling away because their life on this earth is lessening. They are losing the ability to control everything physical, and in many cases losing hold mentally as well. One caregiver wrote, "Boy, do I miss my husband and the way things used to be. Feeling sorry…lonely. I keep saying that my husband's friends have gone away, but I'm realizing that I don't have anyone either. It's probably easier for him because I don't think he notices."

Another one said, "We grieve for the way things were, how our loved ones were, and for the dreams with them that are shattered. Parkinson's just sucks."

Still another put it this way, "It is so very hard to lose them one day at a time.".

And another: "So true…I also see my husband with Parkinson's changing into someone else day by day. It does feel lonely."

I felt anticipatory grief acutely during the years before his death, especially the final five years. However, for me, the grief since his death has been easier than I expected. It has been different than I expected and different than the anticipatory grief, but easier.

Friends, Family, and Clergy

Our support system is critical in the progression of any degenerative disease, and that includes the above-mentioned groups, as well as physicians. The only reason physicians are not listed is because we see them seldom, and even less as our loved one becomes less mobile. But other people are necessary, both for the patient and caregiver.

We were among the many who passed through the worst of Parkinson's during the pandemic of COVID-19. Carlton was placed under hospice care in March of 2020, just as we entered lockdown. At first, the hospice employees didn't even come to the house for fear of spreading germs, and soon after they came the first time, one of the workers came down with COVID, and Carlton had to be tested, along with all other patients in their care.

One of the reasons I have talked about developing a good support system and keeping our friends and family close is due to this experience. During lockdown and in the months following when no one knew how transmissible COVID really was, our friends and family still called consistently, and they came to visit. They were willing to stay six-plus feet away on our outside back patio, or when the weather did not cooperate, they would stay nearly ten feet away inside the house and wear a mask. We were so thankful for their sacrifice in doing this because it kept us from feeling isolated and lonely. We needed their support and encouragement, and they were there to give it.

However, there are friends and/or family who did not come for various reasons. Some just could not bear to see their loved one or friend wasting away from this disease. And that is the unvarnished truth.

At this stage we caregivers are most active in letting them go. That was one of the most difficult things for me. Whether it was cleaning up after him (which was not pleasant), getting up many times during the night to help him get to the bathroom, or picking him up when he had fallen, all of these tasks were inconvenient for me. Nevertheless, watching him "waste away" was painful, and it hurt my heart. He was losing weight rapidly (another indication that he was a good fit for hospice care). As I helped him in the shower, my heart cried because I realized each time that he was thinner. His ribs were showing. He was truly wasting away right before my eyes.

We are all aware that Parkinson's disease is degenerative. He was never going to recover from it, nor would it ever go into remission. Yes, he had some days that were better than others for the first nineteen years or so, but he would never be healed. We do pray that one day there will be a cure for PD, but it is not available at this moment.

Visits from friends and family can be beneficial to all involved with a little preparation. When inviting them, be sure to communicate that your loved one tires easily, and a short visit is better than one that would leave them exhausted. Sometimes people don't know how to leave gracefully, so when they have been there long enough, we can just lean forward in our chair and say, "We are so glad you could come visit today. Would you like to come back in a week or so? We would be glad to have you again." We might even stand at that point. These verbal and non-verbal cues graciously communicate that the visit has been long enough.

In previous chapters we have mentioned our faith community. And as this disease progresses, it becomes more important to have conversations with our loved one about their final wishes, along with their faith. The hope that we gain from our faith is critical as our loved one approaches the end of their life.

We talked about death and dying and funerals and cemeteries many times over the last five years of Carlton's life. I tried to write down everything he wanted and everything he said, and I asked him countless questions. If he wanted to talk about it, I listened and took notes. I also asked our pastors to come to the house to talk with us, especially when we accepted hospice care. The chaplain from the hospice company also came to the house several times, and he spoke with Carlton about his faith. He was kind and compassionate and very skilled at asking questions without judgment or bias. We were very thankful for his visits as well as those from our pastors.

Dementia

According to the definition on the **AARP website**, dementia is "a decline in mental function that is usually irreversible." It causes "chronic **memory loss**, personality changes or impaired reasoning." Many PD patients experience dementia, and it can manifest itself at any time during this journey. One friend of ours had dementia as a first symptom. He was a pastor, and he kept losing his place during his sermons and repeating entire pages. That was the first clue that there was something wrong. However, for many the dementia comes about later in the progression.

A staple in our home was a small dry-erase board. Every morning I wrote the day of the week in large letters at the top of the board. (Some of our friends adopted this same practice, and they also added the date.) Under that, I listed the events planned for that day in chronological order with their times. On special occasions, birthdays, anniversaries, and holidays, I decorated the border of the board using colored markers for fun. Carlton enjoyed that, and the list kept him from asking about our schedule many times in one day. When he did ask, I could walk to the board and point to the answer to his question. Or I could pretend I was reading it for the first time to add a little levity into the conversation.

One of the first ways we might notice dementia in a Parkinson's patient is their inability to make connections between people or the inability to understand how people are connected to places and events. While watching television, Carlton would sometimes forget how characters within a particular show are related, or when presented with new ones, he would think it was a completely different show instead of understanding how they fit into the current situation. This happened off and on for the last five years of his life, but with increasing frequency as time went on.

Another common occurrence was his lack of direction when we were riding in the car. Sometimes he would insist that I should turn left to get to a particular destination when it was really to the right. Problem solving and executive functioning also become impaired. Another thing we noticed was that the order we did things was interrupted because Carlton forgot what should come next.

Sometimes I would say, "It's time to get dressed to go to our daughter's house." He would nod in the affirmative, but then just stand there. Sometimes I needed to say, "Let's go to our bedroom to change your clothes." Often, he would walk into the bedroom and just stand there. I would have to give the next instructions like, "Come over here and sit down, and I'll put on your shoes and socks." The inability to know what comes next in order is part of executive functioning, which diminishes with dementia.

Making decisions became a huge problem. I first noticed this when asking him simple questions like, "What would you like for lunch?" He could not think of any lunch choices. So, then I realized he needed some suggestions. At that point I would list all the combinations we had in our house, which worked for a while. Later on, however, he couldn't even choose from a list, so I gave him only two choices. He could handle deciding between those two for a while—until he just couldn't. He would just freeze. That prompted me to make the decision for him, realizing that he had no preferences anymore, and his brain just couldn't make choices.

Perhaps the saddest part of his mental deterioration for me was that time when he couldn't remember how to turn to sit in a chair. Several times I would help him walk to his lift chair, and when he got close enough to it, he would turn a full 360 degrees before sitting. Sometimes he would even just stand there after that full turn. I would say, "It's okay to sit now," and then gently press him backwards to sit.

The **Parkinsons.org** website is a wealth of information on cognitive changes and other areas of life with Parkinson's. I bookmarked it as one of my "go-to" websites. This cognitive decline does not occur in all PD patients. On the other hand, with some it is the very first symptom that can mask Parkinson's since the doctor is focused on the dementia.

Chapter Four
Hospice Care

Even though chronic illness has a profound impact on life, people adapt to it over time. Sometimes in the back of their minds they even believe that by following their doctor's orders and taking medications on time, one day they will return to health. However, with a degenerative disease, it is understood that one's condition will continue to get worse, and the day may eventually come when the doctor recommends hospice care.

Facing mortality can be daunting, but doing so can foster a better outcome because the true problem is being addressed. At this time of life (and any time, for that matter), it is crucial to aim for the outcome that provides the best quality of life. Determining personal short- and long-term life goals with loved ones can help make this decision-making process easier.

How does the doctor decide if a patient is ready for hospice care? A patient must meet certain criteria to be eligible for this type of care. With a degenerative disease, it is understood that eventually our loved one will become totally dependent. And as they become weaker, there is a point at which hospice could be right for the patient and caregiver. We transitioned to hospice care as much for my benefit as for my husband's. When caring for him became detrimental to my health, I needed help.

In the past few years, the parameters for hospice eligibility have changed. The expected amount of time a patient has left is no longer a major determinant of eligibility. Now the criteria includes the severity of the illness, such as the level of their mobility, and how well that person can perform normal or required daily activities. According to Vitas.com (of Vitas Healthcare), they check for the following signs:

- Rapid progression to wheelchair or bed-bound
- Barely intelligible to unintelligible speech
- Need for puréed foods
- Need for major assistance with eating and personal care, or total dependence on others for these activities

There are many myths surrounding the hospice philosophy such as "Hospice is for people who only have a few days left," or "Hospice means giving up on life." These ideas cannot be further from the truth. Hospice can often allow for a better quality of life and more effective symptom reduction. Many people with chronic conditions suffer from pain, nausea, constipation, insomnia, etc. Part of the beauty of the philosophy of hospice is that the staff works tirelessly to keep the patient comfortable. They strive to manage these annoying symptoms, whereas in traditional healthcare, the symptoms must be tolerated while the treatment of the diagnosed disease is the focus.

Another piece that needs to be evaluated is the burden placed on loved ones to care for the patient's daily needs. Typically, patients in this position are being cared for by an adult who may also have debilitating health problems, or who needs to work full-time. Both situations make it difficult for these loved ones to provide needed physical care for the patient while caring for the home, and perhaps even working an outside job. If this is the case, then hospice can provide help in some of these areas, such as personnel to bathe the patient or provide supportive equipment and supplies. Medicare and/or a hospice company can provide much of the typical medical equipment needed, along with supplies for incontinence, skin care, and other conditions. This relieves the family of the financial burden that often comes with caring for someone with a chronic condition.

Some families elect for their loved one to remain in the home and receive hospice care in comfortable, familiar surroundings. By selecting this option, inpatient care can occasionally be used as respite care for a short period of time, or it can be a short-term solution when the patient's symptoms become too difficult to manage by the home caregiver.

Others choose inpatient hospice services that can provide round-the-clock care for the patient in a long-term care facility or an assisted living community. These decisions should be made by the entire close family considering the welfare of everyone involved. There are pros and cons of both home hospice and a hospice facility, and each family must discuss these alternatives openly and honestly.

All through this caregiving process, one of our goals has been to keep our loved one comfortable, and at no time is this more important than when mobility becomes more challenging. That is the main goal of hospice. At this season of life, no one is trying to "heal" our loved one. We are beyond that. Instead, we are all focused on keeping our loved one clean, comfortable, and calm.

Here are some typical benefits of hospice care:

1. The chaplain, social worker, CNA, and nurse make scheduled visits to the home and are available by phone to answer questions.

2. Hospice personnel are trained for "end of life" issues, and they are a comfort during this sensitive time. I found them to also be helpful when talking with other family members about what to expect as my husband transitioned.

3. As professionals, the hospice staff will work to provide equipment needed for comfort such as a transfer board, pillows to prevent bedsores, a wedge to keep the patient upright, oxygen, hospital bed, etc.

4. The staff will increase the frequency of visits when it becomes necessary. This was of great comfort and encouragement to me.

5. During their visits, they know what questions to ask to recognize failing health. As they repeat their questions with each visit, it is easy to see that their goal is to be aware of the rate of decline.

6. They can advise about fall prevention (such as when transferring from chair to bed to chair), and their suggestions make difficult tasks easier because of their experience.

7. The care received will help keep our loved one out of the hospital as much as possible, which is crucial for Parkinson's patients.

There may be a time when a hospital visit is necessary (especially not connected to Parkinson's Disease.) At that time, it would be wise to listen to the hospice staff since they have been watching the progress of our loved one. The patient may be taken OFF hospice care while in the hospital but can then come back on to hospice care when leaving the hospital.

When our loved one declines and develops a new symptom or problem, the hospice staff will do everything in their power to ease that symptom and make the patient comfortable. That is their main goal.

When you feel the need for significant help in caring for your loved one, speak with your physician about the possibility of hospice care. They may have a provider that they recommend, and that is a good place to begin your search for the right company. However, it is advisable to interview two to three companies whenever possible, making sure to write down what they promise to do. It is important to hold them to the promises they make.

These questions are important to ask in an interview with a prospective hospice company:

1. How can you tell if your loved one is ready for this?

2. What does this really mean for them?

3. What services do you offer, and can we opt out of some?

4. What about their medications?

5. What about our doctors?

6. Do you offer in-home physical therapy?

7. What medical equipment are we eligible for?

8. What do I do in an emergency? Call 911?

9. What if we do not "get along" with the CNA or nurse you send?

10. Can we still travel out of town?

11. What is the cost of your services to us?

12. Does the spouse need to remain home while your employees are here?

13. Is there a CNA available to come on the weekends as well?

14. What happens when my loved one passes? Should I call 911 then?

As caregivers our job is shifting again, and we must be the advocates for our loved ones to the hospice company. They will count on us to know and inform them when we need medications and supplies, and on occasion we must be the squeaky wheel when our loved one is not receiving the services they have promised. (Remember that the hospice company is being paid well to care for our loved one. Let's insist that they provide what has been promised.)

We did encounter one disturbing problem with the hospice system. (This might not be true for every company, but it was true of the ones we used.) When contracting with hospice, we agreed that my husband would not go to his regular physicians again. This was true specifically of his primary care doctor and his neurologist. Their logic was that we were no longer seeking a cure or further treatment for Parkinson's disease, so we no longer needed our neurologist. After twenty-plus years of relying on our neurologist for support and information, this was a huge shift in our thinking.

Regarding my husband's primary care doctor, there was no need for her services again. The hospice company had their own physician who was now in charge of our case. We never met this doctor, which was also strange for us. The nurse who came to visit was tasked with reporting everything to the doctor. It was the nurse who observed my husband, assessed the changes she saw in him, and recommended any medication changes or procedures to the doctor. She sometimes called the doctor while at our house when the situation warranted it.

The disturbing part in all of this was the huge shift in mindset, purpose, procedure, and personnel. It took me a month to understand and redirect my thinking. All of this made sense to me as I remembered the change in philosophy of hospice care as compared to the typical neurologist's visit. We were not focused on curing or improving Carlton's condition. We were now focused on comfort and care.

Hospice care provides us with hope for a dignified and comfortable life when we need it the most. I pray that your experience with them will be as positive as ours was.

Transitioning

From the moment we received the diagnosis of PD, I wondered how my husband would die because Parkinson's by itself is not fatal. According to one **Parkinson's disease website**, most PD patients die from aspirational pneumonia or the result of an injury from falling. However, many coroners write "Parkinson's disease" on the death certificate as the cause of death if the patient has this diagnosis, and they do not look any further.

Even though I had read that website and knew that information, that didn't tell me exactly how it would happen. I assumed he would get sick, go to the hospital, and die there a few days later. But I did not know what would propel us to the hospital.

During our time under hospice care, with each visit from the nurse, it was obvious that my husband's condition was declining. I would often ask the nurse what she was seeing. Sometimes the caregiver is so close to the situation that it's hard to tell how the loved one is changing, but then at other times we see it acutely. The nurse used the term "wasting away" to describe what we were witnessing. He lost nearly a hundred pounds over the last eighteen months, going from the two hundred pounds he weighed most of our married life to 106 pounds. When he died, he was a shell of his former self.

He got weaker by the day, and even when he was not walking, he became so weak he could not even stand alone to be transferred from one chair to another. His appetite declined until he was barely eating half a cup of food per day, and he was drinking only about twelve ounces per day.

At this point in his life, he was talking very little, and he did not ask any questions. That was a huge shift for him since he was always curious about everything. He was no longer interested in our finances, in our children and grandchildren, or in our schedule for the day. It seemed as if he needed all his energy just to stay alive. There was no reserve.

On the last Tuesday of his life, our CNA, Franck, was here to give him a shower. After he got him into the shower, Franck called to me to come help. When I got to the bathroom, I could see that Carlton had fainted in the shower while sitting on the shower chair. I helped Franck hold him as we woke him up, and together we got him out of the shower and into the wheelchair. It took both of us to get him dried and dressed at that point.

Franck told me that he had just had his last shower. We would have to switch to bed baths after this. During this ordeal I noticed what looked like bruising all over his back, and I asked Franck about it. He told me that it was the blood settling, normal for this stage. The website that was a great resource for me at this time was https://hospicefoundation.org/Hospice-Care/Signs-of-Approaching-Death . Since he was going to stay mostly in bed from that point on, we arranged for the hospice company to move his hospital bed from his bedroom into the family room so he wouldn't be alone.

Two days later, our good friends came to visit. He has Parkinson's, and his wife is a fellow caregiver. Carlton was pleased, but he didn't talk much. They stayed only a short while, and as they left, the husband asked Carlton to give him one word for the day. Carlton replied, "Donut!" That was in reference to our earlier conversation, and it was the last word we remember Carlton speaking.

Later that night he slipped into a light coma where he remained off and on for the next five days. He did not eat during that time, but we did give him some medication and sips of liquid. At times he was agitated and fretful in his sleep, so the hospice nurse wanted to give him a small dose of Ativan and morphine to calm him. I resisted these drugs at first, but then I realized that he was leaving this world. He was going to a better place. All along I had been praying for these three things:

1. A peaceful passing

2. The gift of dying at home in his own bed and surroundings

3. No pain at the end of his life

After thinking it over, I realized that the nurse's suggestion would bring those exact results. The medication they gave him was for his comfort and ease. They placed the liquid right inside his mouth with a spoon or syringe, and it calmed him, allowing him to rest. The dosage was not an exact science, which was a bit disconcerting, but I trusted the nurses about this. At this point they were coming every day, and sometimes twice a day.

Our older daughter, Margie, was with me during these last five days, and that was a great comfort. We talked to him often, cried at his bedside, prayed with him, sang to him, and I even played the piano for him. He was peaceful, and we were thankful for that.

We constantly watched his breathing. Sometimes he would stop for a matter of seconds, and then start breathing again. We had read that this might happen, and we should not worry. But we noticed that the time between breaths was increasing. On that last night there was a long time of not breathing, but then when the breath came again, it was short and fast. I felt the change in him, and I sensed that the end of his life was near.

On the fourth night, I finally went to bed around midnight, and Margie slept in the chair beside his bed. She was so close that she could reach her hand through the railing and touch his hand. She fell asleep sometime around 2:00 a.m., and when she awoke at 4:30 a.m., he was not breathing. When she touched him, his skin was cold. She knew he had slipped from this world into the next, so she came and woke me.

Our first thought was that we were so thankful that he was no longer sick. Thankful that we had been part of something beautiful. Thankful that God had heard our prayers, the three prayers mentioned above. Carlton was free. Our tears and grief were the result of our loss, not his. He had been a huge presence in our lives, and his passing left a giant hole in our family. The last twenty-three years had been centered around him—his care, his memories, his life, his well-being. Our caregiving came to a screeching halt on that morning.

Because he was under hospice care, we called the hospice office right away, and they sent the nurse to the house. After the nurse pronounced his death, she called the mortuary that had been prearranged just a few weeks ago. She also made the arrangements for the hospice company to pick up the medical equipment when it was convenient for me.

Even at that time it seemed to me that Carlton's transition from this world to the next was beautifully organic. It was nearly seamless, and it seemed so natural. There were tense moments when he was asleep for those last days because I fully expected him to wake up and need to eat or drink. I didn't know what was expected of me during that time, so I talked with Nurse Rachel and our CNA, Franck. They assured me that this was natural and normal, and Carlton would show us what would come next.

I will be eternally grateful for our hospice company and the employees with whom we interacted. They were professional, yet empathetic. They were caring, yet clinical. They were with us every step of the way, and I'm so glad we didn't have to go through this time alone.

After the Passing

After the passing and the body has been removed, there are a million things to do. The exact order of the first few notifications is very important so that no one gets their feelings hurt.

You might consider this order for notifications:

1. Immediate family, which may include children, siblings, parents, and even pastors. Be sure this inner circle is notified first. Warning: Decide who will post on social media, including exactly what will be said, and then allow everyone else to share that post. This is the best way to control the narrative.

2. Close friends and next layer of family, which may include cousins, aunts, and uncles, etc.

3. Casual friends who might not see it on social media.

4. Doctors and co-workers, professional friends.

The next big decisions involve the following:

1. Will there be a service?

2. When and where?

3. Who will participate?

4. Who will attend—public or family only?

5. Will the body be cremated or not?

6. If the body is cremated, what to do with the ashes?

7. If not cremated, where will the body be buried?

If you have an attorney, call them in the first one to three days. Ours set up a Zoom call with me and explained what to do about these issues:

1. Social Security

2. Insurance companies

3. Medicare

4. Bank accounts

5. Accountant

6. Other agencies or official entities that should be notified

Chapter Five
What I Learned From Caregiving

When we get to the other side and the caregiving is over, it is good to look back for a minute. As in most experiences, there are positive and negative takeaways. We always hope the positives outweigh the negatives to register an overall gain for the time and effort spent, especially when many days were unpleasant, and it seemed as if our tasks would never end.

C. S. Lewis once said, "Adventures are never fun while you're having them." Caregiving was an adventure—an unplanned one. Sometimes it was fun, but many times it was hard work and felt like walking through a dark forest. We didn't ask for it, but neither did our loved one. I mentioned that truism to God in those exact words on several occasions when the days were long, and the nights were longer. It felt good to be able to say that to God; however, I tried not to mention that to Carlton. But it was an adventure we were traveling together through uncharted territory.

In the months since my husband passed into heaven in May of 2021, I can see many things more clearly in retrospect. The big picture is much more evident in hindsight, which has 20/20 vision. Here are some positive things that have come from that adventure:

Positive Lesson #1

I learned patience in several different ways during those twenty-three years. When Carlton used to freeze, especially in doorways, I was mortified when strangers had to wait until he could move again. I was very embarrassed. But I soon realized that I just had to be patient because there was absolutely nothing I could do to help him in those circumstances. I had to exercise that same patience often when his condition worsened and his mobility decreased. Everything he did became slower and slower, so I had to learn to match that speed. During this time, I had a good friend who constantly reminded me to stop and imagine how my husband must feel in these situations. He asked me to put myself in Carlton's shoes. How must it feel to know that your condition would certainly worsen? How would I feel knowing that I would become slower and slower and less able to move by the day?

Positive Lesson #2

I learned that many problems cannot be completely solved. Instead, we might have to find a workable solution, like a band-aid, that would allow us to live WITH the problem, instead of conquering it. It had always been my habit to solve problems. My career as a teacher of mathematics was filled with solving equations, solving story problems, and focusing on the answer. But I could not fix my husband. I could not heal his Parkinson's. I could not even totally prevent him from falling, as much as I tried. Later in the course of the disease, I could not prevent his constipation and diarrhea, even though I tried every home remedy possible. There were many problems I could not solve, so I had to be content to learn how to help him live comfortably with the problem. That was humbling, but it was reality.

Positive Lesson #3

I also learned that I was strong. There were several things I had to do that caused me to feel like a fish out of water. They were totally out of my comfort zone. One involved taking care of my husband's Foley catheter. I am not medically trained, nor to do I wish to be. But I had to figure out how to use his catheter. The nurse at the urologist's office gave me two minutes of instructions, but when we got home, I felt totally overwhelmed and could not remember anything she had said. So, it was YouTube to the rescue! I watched a video on how to change the bags and care for his catheter, and that was how I learned. The great thing about the videos is that you can watch them multiple times, stop them whenever you want, and rewind them to see what you missed.

I could do this, even though I was not perfect. And as we all must do at times, I had to accept my imperfections. But I also realized that I could succeed in accomplishing my three main goals—to keep my husband safe and clean and happy. Sometime during caregiving, I actually wrote down those three goals because all the other things in life paled in importance to them. Seeing those on paper allowed me to forgive myself for other things that were squeezed out of my life, like feeling the need to decorate for every season, wanting to plant new flowers each season, planning a social life for us, trying new recipes, and redecorating the house to replace things that were wearing out. I would have done all those things in a normal time of life. But watching your loved one's physical condition deteriorate daily is not normal for most people.

Besides doing the physical labor of caring for my husband, I learned that I could make decisions for us, even when I had to do them alone. One of the worst parts of Parkinson's is the cognitive decline. This is different for everyone, but we should expect cognitive problems as the disease progresses. Therefore, we must make the best use of the early years after diagnosis to make the major decisions concerning "end of life" and estate planning together. For many caregivers, including myself, the day will likely come when the major decisions are made unilaterally because our loved one cannot think clearly enough to help.

Positive Lesson #4

I learned that there is a time in all of our lives when we need help. And I certainly did. Not only was I providing caregiving for my husband, but I was also doing it during the COVID-19 pandemic. The United States went on lockdown in March of 2020, which is the same month that my husband went under hospice care. We were confined to our home for several weeks, which meant that some of the normal pressures of life were eased for us. We were not the only ones who were confined. It was everyone. That meant as he got worse and we stayed home, the rest of the country was also staying home. In many ways we thrived under the lockdown order.

I will be eternally grateful to the friends and family who called to check on us daily and even Zoomed with us. At first, he would sit beside me on the Zoom calls and speak when someone addressed him. But eventually that was too difficult for him. Several friends came to our house to visit him/us during that time, and they sat six to eight feet away from us to keep safe. They did not want us to feel alone, even during a pandemic. On many occasions they brought food and puzzles and flowers and gifts. Their efforts encouraged and supported us during the entire ordeal. We really needed "all hands on deck" during that time, and thankfully, they were there for us.

But at the same time, we cannot overlook the negative effects of our time of isolation due to the pandemic. Here are a few of those:

First, I felt loneliness more acutely than ever before. I felt that I was caring for my husband totally by myself, and I was. At first even the hospice workers did not come into the house, and I felt very isolated. Gradually they entered the house with masks, for which we were very thankful. We were still alone during the long hours of the remainder of the day and night. The isolation was painful at times, and the weight of the pandemic was depressing.

But thankfully we came through it by leaning into our friends, family, and faith. Our friends and pastors were faithful to call and visit, and the time spent with them was uplifting and encouraging.

In 2018, both of our daughters lived in other states, but noticing that Carlton's condition was obviously declining, our older daughter and family moved to our city to be near us and help us. We will be forever grateful to them for seeing and meeting our needs. This meant that they were close at hand during the pandemic and through the final days of his life. We are equally thankful for our other daughter and family who live in Kansas. They stayed in touch almost daily and made several trips to see us in the last years of his life. We are blessed with family, friends, and pastors who were God's gifts to us during this time.

Second, my personal health and well-being took a hit. Near the end of Carlton's life, it took so much energy and time to care for him that I had nothing left for myself. I neglected my own health by skipping check-ups and dental cleanings because we were afraid of contracting COVID, or because it was so much work to get a sitter for Carlton. It became easier to just stay home. Thankfully, this did not last long.

Regrets

I have a few regrets from this time. Thankfully, there are only a few, and I have forgiven myself and moved on. Sharing them here is part of being honest and vulnerable, and perhaps by sharing them you will have even fewer regrets.

Early after receiving the Parkinson's diagnosis, I promised my husband that I would keep him at home until he passed away. He did not ask for this as far as I remember, and the details of the conversation are fuzzy in my mind now, except for the promise I made. Truthfully, I wish I had not made that promise. We cannot see the future, so we don't know how dependent our loved one will be, and we don't know what our physical condition at that time will be. I'm glad I could keep him at home, but things could have turned out differently, and I might have had to break my promise.

Also, I wish I had taken better care of myself during his illness. I tried to do that, and I heard many medical professionals and others admonish me to do that, but real life just seemed to get in the way. Sometimes I just couldn't do one more thing in a day. For the last several years of his life I did not sleep well. He would fall out of bed, which woke me up, or he would need to get up three or four times on many nights, and I would struggle to get back to sleep.

So, my nights were broken up, and I couldn't get a good night's sleep. I wish I had asked for help more often. That would have better preserved my physical and mental status. As I became more tired, I became less patient. It was a vicious circle.

Enough

Sometimes while caring for someone with a degenerative disease, we have occasion to doubt ourselves. To think we are the wrong person for the job. To think God must have made a mistake—surely someone else could do this better. After all, we are so imperfect.

Our loved one is not getting better. (We knew they wouldn't, but somehow we expected them to improve since we are giving them such good care!) And there are times when they do seem better. They will have good days in between the bad ones. It really doesn't help that it seems we are on a roller coaster.

When a new symptom appears, we are tempted to cry, "Great! One more thing for me to do. Something new to worry about. Don't I have enough symptoms on my plate already?" And there will be more symptoms soon, and after that—more symptoms. That is the way of a degenerative disease.

And just when we think we have reached the end of a particular problem, it flares back up again. The most annoying problem for us during Parkinson's was the constipation/diarrhea rollercoaster. As soon as we licked the constipation, it seemed like Carlton would have one good day, and then diarrhea would hit. It was a constant pendulum swing. This was his Achilles heel, so it seemed.

Others may find falling to be a problem. And once you have removed all obstacles, found good shoes for them to wear, placed the walker or cane close by, they might go a day or two with no falls, and then they fall and break a bone, causing more problems for everyone.

As caregivers we doubt ourselves and think it might be our fault. *Did I leave him alone too long? Did I leave that box in the way that he tripped over? Did I forget to remind him to use the walker? I must be a bad caregiver.*

All that self-doubt creeps into our minds, and the questioning begins all over. Instead of listening to those negative voices, it helps to ask ourselves just one simple question: *Did I do my best to help him/her?* If the answer is yes, we must push away every negative thought and remember that we are enough. We are doing all we can in each situation. We are not perfect, we are not medically trained, and we are not super-human. We do the best we can. We are enough.

Let's do our best, and then we can hold our head up high and be proud of the work we have done to help our loved one. We have sacrificed our time and in some cases our careers, and we have given or are giving all we have.

WAYS TO CONTACT CHERYL

Visit her website – hopeforparkinsons.net

Email her – cherylcaregiver71@gmail.com

Read her blog – www.parkinsonscaregivernet.wordpress.com

ORDER INFORMATION

Do you know someone with Parkinson's Disease?
This book would make a great gift.

To order additional copies of this book or
other inspiration books visit Amazon.

www.ingramcontent.com/pod-product-compliance
Lightning Source LLC
LaVergne TN
LVHW051956060526
838201LV00059B/3673